Concussion: A Patient's Guide to Understanding and Coping

Dr Ioannis Mavroudis

TABLE OF CONTENTS

Preface

In recent years, there has been an increased awareness and concern about the effects of concussions on the human brain. This book is a valuable resource for patients who have experienced a concussion or for those who want to learn more about this condition.

The book is written in a clear and accessible language, making it easy for patients to understand the causes, symptoms, and consequences of a concussion. It provides tips and techniques to help patients manage their symptoms and recovery process. The book also includes real-life examples and case studies that illustrate the impact of concussions on different individuals and their families.

One of the most important aspects of this book is that it emphasizes the importance of seeking medical attention if you suspect that you or someone you know has a concussion. The book is not intended to replace medical opinion or to be used for diagnosis or treatment. However, it can help patients to better understand the condition, ask informed questions and make informed decisions about their care.

The book also includes information on the long-term effects of repeated concussions, and the importance of taking concussions seriously, even if the symptoms seem mild. It also covers the importance of prevention and steps that can be taken to reduce the risk of concussions in sports, work, and everyday life.

Overall, this book is an essential guide for anyone who has experienced a concussion or wants to learn more about this condition. It provides valuable information and tools to help patients understand and manage their concussion and ultimately improve their recovery process.

— Dr Ioannis Mavroudis MD, PhD, Consultant Neurologist & Senior Lecturer in Neurology

Concussion: A Patient's Guide to Understanding and Coping

Introduction

The Human Brain

The human brain is a complex and fascinating organ that controls all of the body's functions, from breathing and heart rate to thoughts and emotions. It is made up of billions of nerve cells, called neurons, which communicate with each other to process information and coordinate the body's activities.

One of the key functions of the brain is to receive and process information from the senses, such as sight, sound, taste, touch, and smell. This information is then used to control the body's movements and responses.

The brain is also responsible for controlling our emotions and thoughts. The cerebral cortex, the brain's outermost layer, is responsible for higher cognitive functions such as reasoning, memory, and decision-making. The limbic system, which is located deep within the brain, is responsible for our emotional responses.

In addition to these functions, the brain also plays a critical role in maintaining our overall health and well-being. It controls important physiological processes such as breathing and heart rate, and it also regulates the release of hormones that play a role in metabolism, growth, and development.

It's important to note that the brain can be affected by various factors such as disease, injury, or certain lifestyle choices, which can lead to changes in brain function. That's why it is important to take care of our brain by engaging in healthy habits such as regular exercise, getting enough sleep, and eating a balanced diet.

Neurons

Neurons are the basic building blocks of the brain and nervous system. They are specialised cells that transmit information throughout the body. Each neuron has a cell body, dendrites, and an axon. The dendrites receive information from other neurons, while the axon sends information to other neurons or to muscles and glands.

When a neuron receives a signal, it generates an electrical impulse that travels down the axon. When this impulse reaches the end of the axon, it triggers the release of chemical neurotransmitters. These neurotransmitters then bind to receptors on the dendrites of other neurons, transmitting the electrical impulse and passing the information along.

This process of transmitting information from one neuron to another is called synaptic transmission. It is the basic mechanism by which neurons communicate with each other, and it is what enables the brain to process information and coordinate the body's activities.

Cognition is the process of acquiring, processing, and using information. It is the ability to think, reason, and remember. In the brain, cognition is a result of the communication between neurons, which work together to process information. The neurons form connections, called synapses, with other neurons, allowing them to transmit information. The more connections a neuron has, the more it can process information, and the more complex the cognition is.

Cognition is a result of the communication and interaction between different areas of the brain. Different regions of the brain are responsible for different cognitive processes, such as perception, attention, memory, and language. When these regions communicate and work together, it enables us to think, reason, and remember.

It's important to note that the brain is plastic and it can change and adapt over time, in response to experiences and learning. So, by keeping our brain active and engaged through reading, solving puzzles, learning new skills, and other mentally stimulating activities, we can help to maintain and improve cognitive function.

The Lobes of the human brain

The frontal lobe is a region of the brain located at the front of the cerebral hemispheres. It is one of the four main lobes of the brain and is the largest of the lobes. It is responsible for a variety of functions, including:

Executive functions: The frontal lobe is responsible for cognitive processes such as planning, decision-making, problem-solving, and organising. It also helps to control impulsivity and inhibit inappropriate responses.

Motor control: The frontal lobe is responsible for controlling movement and coordination. It helps to plan and execute movements, as well as control the fine movements of the hands and fingers.

Emotion and personality: The frontal lobe is responsible for regulating emotions and plays a role in personality development. It is also involved in social behaviour and communication.

Speech and language: The frontal lobe is responsible for producing speech and understanding language. Damage to the frontal lobe can result in difficulty with language and speech production, known as aphasia.

Working memory: The frontal lobe is responsible for maintaining information in the mind for brief periods of time, known as working memory.

Damage to the frontal lobe can lead to a variety of problems, such as difficulty with executive functions, motor control, and emotional regulation. Trauma, stroke, and neurodegenerative disorders can all cause damage to the frontal lobe. Treatment and therapy can help to compensate for any deficits caused by damage to the frontal lobe.

Temporal lobe

The temporal lobe is a region of the brain located on the sides of the cerebral hemispheres, beneath the lateral sulcus (also known as the Sylvian fissure). It is one of the four main lobes of the brain and is involved in a variety of functions, including:

Auditory processing: The temporal lobe is responsible for processing sound and is involved in the perception of speech and music. Damage to the temporal lobe can result in difficulty with hearing and understanding speech, known as auditory processing disorder.

Memory: The temporal lobe is involved in the formation of long-term memories. It is responsible for the consolidation of information from short-term memory into long-term memory and plays a role in the recall of memories. Damage to the temporal lobe can result in difficulty with memory, known as amnesia.

Language: The temporal lobe is involved in the understanding of language and the ability to use language. Damage to the temporal lobe can result in difficulty with language, known as aphasia.

Perception: The temporal lobe is responsible for processing visual information and is involved in the perception of objects and scenes. Damage to the temporal lobe can result in difficulty with visual perception, known as agnosia.

Emotion: The temporal lobe is involved in the processing of emotional information and the regulation of emotion. Damage to the temporal lobe can result in difficulty with emotional regulation, known as emotional dysregulation.

Damage to the temporal lobe can be caused by a variety of factors such as trauma, stroke, or neurodegenerative disorders such as Alzheimer's disease. Treatment and therapy can help to compensate for any deficits caused by damage to the temporal lobe.

Parietal lobe

The parietal lobe is a region of the brain located at the top and back of the cerebral hemispheres, behind the frontal and temporal lobes. It is one of the four main lobes of the brain and is responsible for a variety of functions, including:

Sensation: The parietal lobe is responsible for processing information from the senses, such as touch, temperature, pain, and pressure. It helps to create a map of the body's sensory receptors, known as the somatosensory cortex. Damage to the parietal lobe can result in difficulty with sensation, known as sensory loss.

Perception: The parietal lobe is responsible for processing visual and auditory information and is involved in the perception of spatial relationships and the identification of objects and their properties. Damage to the parietal lobe can result in difficulty with perception, known as agnosia.

Motor control: The parietal lobe is involved in the planning and execution of movement, as well as the control of fine movements of the hands and fingers. Damage to the parietal lobe can result in difficulty with motor control, known as apraxia.

Maths and spatial reasoning: The parietal lobe is responsible for mathematical and spatial reasoning and is involved in the understanding of numbers and mathematical operations. Damage to the parietal lobe can result in difficulty with math and spatial reasoning, known as acalculia and agnosia.

Damage to the parietal lobe can be caused by a variety of factors such as trauma, stroke, or neurodegenerative disorders such as Alzheimer's disease. Treatment and therapy can help to compensate for any deficits caused by damage to the parietal lobe.

Occipital lobe

The occipital lobe is a region of the brain located at the back of the cerebral hemispheres, behind the parietal and temporal lobes. It is one of the four main lobes of the brain and is responsible for processing visual information, which is one of its most important functions. The main functions of the occipital lobe include:

Vision: The occipital lobe is responsible for processing visual information and is involved in the interpretation of images and the ability to see. Damage to the occipital lobe can result in visual disturbances such as visual hallucinations, blind spots, and loss of vision.

Colour vision: The occipital lobe is responsible for the perception of colour, and damage to this region may cause colour blindness or difficulty distinguishing between colours.

Depth perception: The occipital lobe is involved in the perception of depth and 3D spatial relationships, which allows us to understand the distance and position of objects in space.

Motion perception: The occipital lobe plays a role in the perception of motion and the ability to track moving objects. Damage to this region may cause difficulty with motion perception.

Damage to the occipital lobe can be caused by a variety of factors such as trauma, stroke, tumours, or neurodegenerative disorders. Treatment and therapy can help to compensate for any deficits caused by damage to the occipital lobe.

Insula of Reil

The insula of Reil, also known as the insula or the insular cortex, is a region of the brain located deep within the lateral sulcus (also known as the Sylvian fissure), between the temporal and frontal lobes. It is a complex and multifaceted area that is involved in a wide range of functions, including:

Interoception: The insula is responsible for the perception of internal body states, such as heart rate, blood pressure, temperature, and pain. It helps to integrate information from various internal organs and the immune system, and is involved in the regulation of homeostasis.

Emotion: The insula is involved in the processing of emotional information, including the perception of emotions in oneself and others, as well as emotional regulation. Damage to the insula can result in difficulty with emotional regulation, known as emotional dysregulation.

Social cognition: The insula is involved in the perception of social cues, such as tone of voice, facial expressions, and body language, and is also involved in empathy and theory of mind. Damage to the insula can result in difficulty with social cognition, known as social dysregulation.

Taste: The insula is involved in the perception of taste and the integration of taste with other sensory information, such as smell and texture. Damage to the insula can result in difficulty with taste, known as dysgeusia.

Motor control: The insula is also involved in the planning and execution of movement, and the control of fine movements of the hand. Damage to the insula can result in difficulty with motor control, known as apraxia.

Damage to the insula can be caused by a variety of factors such as stroke, trauma, and neurodegenerative disorders. Treatment and therapy can help to compensate for any deficits caused by damage to the insula.

Thalamus and Hypothalamus

The thalamus and hypothalamus are two important structures located in the brain that play key roles in a variety of functions.

The thalamus is a large, egg-shaped structure located in the centre of the brain, and acts as a relay station for incoming sensory information. It receives and processes information from the senses, such as touch, vision, and hearing, and sends it to the appropriate areas of the brain for further processing. The thalamus also plays a role in the regulation of consciousness, sleep, and arousal. Damage to the thalamus can result in disturbances in sensation, movement, and consciousness.

The hypothalamus is a small, almond-shaped structure located beneath the thalamus, and plays a key role in the regulation of the body's internal environment. It helps to control various physiological functions, such as body temperature, hunger, thirst, and blood pressure, and also plays a role in emotions, motivation, and the regulation of the endocrine system. The hypothalamus also controls the autonomic nervous system, which regulates the body's unconscious functions, such as heart rate and breathing. Damage to the hypothalamus can result in a wide range of disorders, including diabetes insipidus, hypothermia, and disorders of the autonomic nervous system.

Both the thalamus and hypothalamus are important structures that play a critical role in maintaining the body's overall balance and homeostasis. Damage to these structures can result in a wide range of disorders and dysfunction.

Chapter 1

CONCUSSION

Mild Traumatic Brain Injury

Definition of concussion

A concussion is a type of brain injury that occurs when the brain is suddenly and violently jolted or shaken inside the skull. This can happen as a result of a blow to the head, such as from a fall or a car accident, or from a sudden, violent movement of the head, such as when playing sports. Concussions can also be caused by a blow to the body that causes the head to move suddenly, such as when a person is punched in the face.

Symptoms of a concussion may include headache, dizziness, confusion, memory problems, nausea, vomiting, and difficulty with balance or coordination. In severe cases, a person with a concussion may lose consciousness. Concussions can range in severity from mild to severe, and treatment will depend on the severity of the injury. In most cases, rest and time are the best remedies for a concussion. However, in severe cases, medical attention may be necessary.

Chapter 2

Biomechanics of traumatic brain injury

Mechanisms of Injury

Traumatic brain injury (TBI) can be caused by a variety of mechanisms, including blunt force trauma, penetrating injury, and acceleration-deceleration forces. The biomechanics of TBI refer to the ways in which these different mechanisms affect the brain and the body.

Blunt force trauma

Blunt force trauma occurs when the head is struck by an object or surface. This can cause the brain to move rapidly inside the skull, leading to injuries such as contusions (bruises) and diffuse axonal injury (tears in the nerve fibers of the brain).

Penetrating injury

Penetrating injuries occur when an object pierces the skull and enters the brain. These injuries can cause more localized damage and are often more severe than blunt force injuries.

Acceleration-deceleration

Acceleration-deceleration forces occur when the head is rapidly accelerated or decelerated. This can cause the brain to move inside the skull, leading to injuries such as coup-contrecoup injuries, where the brain is bruised on the side of impact and then on the opposite side as it rebounds against the skull.

Shear injury

Shear injuries occur due to the brain moving in different directions than the skull, causing injury to the nerve fibers of the brain.

The biomechanics of TBI can also be affected by the individual's age, sex, and overall health, and the severity of the injury can vary widely. Understanding the biomechanics of TBI is important for developing effective treatments and preventions.

It's important to note that TBI is a complex injury that affects multiple systems and functions, and the biomechanical understanding of the injury is just one aspect of it. Other factors such as brain chemistry, inflammation, and genetics also play a role in the injury and recovery process.

Chapter 3

Pathophysiology of concussion

Pathogenetic mechanisms

The exact pathophysiology of concussion is not fully understood, but it is thought to involve several different mechanisms.

One of these mechanisms is mechanical deformation of brain tissue, which can cause stretching or tearing of neurons and blood vessels. This can lead to inflammation and swelling in the brain, as well as changes in the levels of neurotransmitters and other chemicals in the brain.

Axons are long, slender projections of nerve cells that transmit electrical signals between the cells. They are responsible for transmitting information from the brain and spinal cord to the rest of the body.

Axonal damage, also known as axonal injury, is a type of injury that occurs when axons are damaged or disrupted. This can occur as a result of a concussion, which is a type of traumatic brain injury that occurs when the brain is jarred or shaken inside the skull.

During a concussion, the brain can be damaged by the impact or by the sudden movement of the head. This can result in a range of symptoms, including atonia, headache, dizziness, nausea, fatigue, and difficulty with memory, concentration, and communication.

In addition to these symptoms, axonal damage can also cause changes in the brain's function. It can disrupt the normal transmission of signals between nerve cells, leading to problems with movement, sensation, and cognition. Axonal damage may also cause inflammation and swelling in the brain, which can further disrupt normal brain function.

Another mechanism that may contribute to concussion is the formation of microhemorrhages, or small bleeds, in the brain. These bleeds can cause additional damage to brain tissue and may contribute to the symptoms of concussion. Microhemorrhages are small, microscopic bleeding in the brain that can occur as a result of a concussion or other traumatic brain injury. They are often too small to be seen on standard brain imaging

tests, but can be detected using specialised techniques such as magnetic resonance imaging (MRI) with susceptibility weighted imaging (SWI).

Microhemorrhages can occur when blood vessels in the brain are damaged or torn by the impact or sudden movement of the head during a concussion. The bleeding can cause inflammation and swelling in the brain, which can disrupt normal brain function.

Microhemorrhages can also lead to the buildup of iron in the brain, which can be toxic to nerve cells. This can result in further damage to the brain and may contribute to the long-term effects of a concussion, such as cognitive impairment, memory loss, and mood changes.

In addition to these mechanical and structural changes, concussion can also affect brain function. It may impair the brain's ability to process and integrate information, as well as its ability to regulate mood and emotion. These functional changes can contribute to the cognitive and emotional symptoms that are often seen with concussion.

One of the most common symptoms of a concussion is difficulty with cognition, which includes processes such as memory, concentration, and decision-making. A person with a concussion may experience difficulty with tasks that require mental effort or concentration, such as reading, writing, or solving problems. They may also have difficulty with memory, both short-term and long-term.

The brain's ability to process information is complex and involves many different areas of the brain. When the brain is injured, it can affect the normal functioning of these areas and lead to cognitive problems.

For example, a concussion can cause damage to the frontal lobe, which is responsible for many cognitive functions such as problem-solving, decision-making, and planning. Damage to the frontal lobe can lead to difficulty with these tasks and may also cause changes in personality and behaviour.

A concussion can also affect the temporal lobe, which is involved in memory and language processing. Damage to the temporal lobe can cause problems with memory and the ability to understand and use language.

In addition to these specific areas of the brain, a concussion can also affect the brain's overall functioning by causing inflammation and swelling, which can further disrupt normal brain function.

Chapter 4

Brief overview of the prevalence and impact of concussion

Epidemiology of concussion

Concussions are relatively common, especially in children and adolescents who are active in sports and other high-energy activities. According to the Centers for Disease Control and Prevention (CDC), an estimated 1.6 to 3.8 million sports- and recreation-related concussions occur each year in the United States. Concussions are also common in car accidents and other types of traumatic events. According to the Centers for Disease Control and Prevention (CDC), in the United States:

Approximately 1.7 million people sustain a concussion each year.

Concussions are most common in children and adolescents, with sports- and recreation-related activities being the leading cause of concussions in this age group.

Concussions account for approximately 10% of all sports-related injuries.

Football, soccer, and basketball are the sports with the highest rates of concussion.

The impact of a concussion can vary widely, depending on the severity of the injury and the individual's age, health, and other factors. In general, most people who experience a concussion will fully recover within a few weeks or months. However, some people may experience long-term symptoms, such as headaches, memory problems, and difficulty with balance or coordination. In rare cases, a severe traumatic brain injury or repetitive concussions can lead to more serious complications, such as bleeding in the brain or an increased risk of developing neurodegenerative conditions such as dementia or Parkinson's disease.

It is important to seek medical attention if you or someone you know experiences a concussion, especially if the person loses consciousness or experiences severe symptoms. Early diagnosis and treatment can help to prevent long-term complications and ensure a full recovery.

Chapter 5

Causes

Common causes of concussion

There are many potential causes of concussion, including:

Falls

A fall from a significant height, such as from a ladder or a rooftop, can cause a concussion. Children and older adults are particularly prone to falls and the resulting concussions. Falls can cause concussions and other types of brain injury. The impact of the fall can cause the brain to be jarred or shaken inside the skull, leading to a concussion. Falls can occur at any age, but they are more common in children and older adults. Falls can also cause other types of brain injuries, such as skull fractures, brain bleeds, and brain swelling. The severity of the injury will depend on the height of the fall and the surface on which the person falls.

Sports and physical activity

Concussions are common in contact sports, such as football and boxing, as well as in high-energy activities such as skateboarding and snowboarding. Sports and other high-energy activities can increase the risk of concussion and other types of brain injury. The impact of a hit, fall, or collision can cause the brain to be jarred or shaken inside the skull, leading to a concussion. Sports and other high-energy activities that carry a high risk of concussion include contact sports, such as football, hockey, and boxing, as well as non-contact sports, such as soccer and basketball.

Traffic accidents

Car accidents are a leading cause of concussions, especially if the person was not wearing a seatbelt at the time of the accident. Traffic accidents, including car accidents, motorcycle accidents, and pedestrian accidents, can cause concussions and other types of brain injuries. The impact of the collision can cause the brain to be jarred or shaken inside the skull, leading to a concussion.

Physical violence

A concussion can result from a punch, kick, or other physical assault. Physical violence, including assault, domestic violence, and child abuse, can cause concussions and other types of brain injury. The impact of the violence can cause the brain to be jarred or shaken inside the skull, leading to a concussion.

Blast injuries

Concussions can be caused by exposure to explosive blasts, such as those that occur in military combat or terrorist attacks. Blasts, including those from explosives or from other sources, such as fireworks or industrial accidents, can cause concussions and other types of brain injuries. The impact of a blast can cause the brain to be jarred or shaken inside the skull, leading to a concussion. Symptoms of a concussion caused by a blast may include headache, dizziness, confusion, memory problems, nausea and vomiting, fatigue, sensitivity to light and noise, sleep disturbances, and mood changes.

Shaken baby syndrome

This type of concussion occurs when a baby is violently shaken, which can cause the brain to move around inside the skull and lead to injury.

It is important to take precautions to prevent concussions, such as wearing a seatbelt, using protective gear when participating in sports or other high-energy activities, and supervising young children to prevent falls. If you or someone you know experiences a concussion, it is important to seek medical attention as soon as possible.

Chapter 6

Risk factors for concussions

There are several factors that can increase the risk of concussion, including:

Age

Children and older adults are more prone to concussions than younger adults.

Participation in sports and other high-energy activities

People who participate in contact sports or other activities that involve high speeds or impacts are at greater risk of concussion.

Previous concussions

People who have had a concussion in the past are at higher risk of experiencing another one.

Substance abuse

Substance abuse, including alcohol abuse, can increase the risk of concussion.

Medical conditions

Certain medical conditions, such as epilepsy, can increase the risk of concussion.

Poor physical condition

People who are in poor physical condition may be more prone to concussion due to weaker muscles and bones.

It is important to be aware of these risk factors and take steps to protect yourself and others from concussion. This may include wearing protective gear when participating in sports or other high-energy activities, avoiding substance abuse, and maintaining good physical condition. If you or someone you know experiences a concussion, it is important to seek medical attention as soon as possible.

Chapter 7

Common symptoms of concussion

Symptomatology

The symptoms of a concussion can vary widely, and may include:

Headache

A headache is the most common symptom of a concussion. It may be mild or severe, and may feel like pressure or a dull ache. Headache may occur as a result of the brain being jarred or shaken inside the skull during the injury. Concussion-related headaches may be described as a pressure sensation or a throbbing pain, and may be accompanied by other symptoms, such as dizziness, nausea, and sensitivity to light and noise. Headaches can range in severity from mild to severe. According to the Centers for Disease Control and Prevention (CDC), approximately 50% of people who sustain a concussion report experiencing a headache as a symptom. The severity and duration of headaches after a concussion can vary depending on a number of factors, including the severity of the concussion, the patient's age and medical history, and other risk factors for headaches. In general, headaches after a concussion tend to be more severe and longer-lasting in those who have a history of headaches or migraines, and in those who have more severe or complicated concussions. Concussion-related headaches may resolve on their own over time, but in some cases, they may persist or become chronic. Chronic headaches after a concussion are known as post-concussion syndrome.

Dizziness

A person with a concussion may feel dizzy or lightheaded, or may have trouble with balance or coordination. Dizziness is a common symptom of concussion, and may occur as a result of the brain being jarred or shaken inside the skull during the injury. According to the Centers for Disease Control and Prevention (CDC), approximately 40% of people who sustain a concussion report experiencing dizziness as a symptom.

The severity and duration of dizziness after a concussion can vary depending on a number of factors, including the severity of the concussion, the patient's age and medical history, and other risk factors for dizziness. In general, dizziness after a concussion tends to be more severe and longer-lasting in those who have a history of dizziness or balance disorders, and in those who have more severe or complicated concussions. Concussion-related dizziness may be described as a sensation of spinning or tilting, and may be accompanied by other symptoms, such as headache, nausea, and difficulty with balance and coordination.

Concussion-related dizziness may resolve on its own over time, but in some cases, it may persist or become chronic. Chronic dizziness after a concussion is known as post-concussion syndrome.

Confusion

A concussion can cause confusion, disorientation, or difficulty thinking clearly. Confusion is a common symptom of concussion, and may occur as a result of the brain being jarred or shaken inside the skull during the injury. Concussion-related confusion may manifest as difficulty with memory, concentration, and decision-making, and may be accompanied by other symptoms, such as headache, dizziness, and fatigue.

Concussion-related confusion may resolve on its own over time, but in some cases, it may persist or become chronic. Chronic confusion after a concussion is known as post-concussion syndrome.

Memory problems

A person with a concussion may have trouble remembering new information or events that occurred around the time of the injury. Memory problems are a common symptom of concussion, and may occur as a result of the brain being jarred or shaken inside the skull during the injury. Concussion-related memory problems may manifest as difficulty with learning new information, recalling past events, or retaining information over time, and may be accompanied by other symptoms, such as headache, dizziness, and confusion. Memory problems, including difficulty with short-term memory, long-term memory, and memory consolidation, are common after a concussion, and according to the Centers for Disease Control and Prevention (CDC), approximately 50% of people who sustain a concussion report experiencing memory problems as a symptom.

Distractibility

Distractibility is a term used to describe the inability to focus or concentrate on a task or activity.

Distractibility can make it difficult to complete tasks or engage in activities that require mental effort or concentration, such as reading, writing, or solving problems. It can also make it difficult to pay attention to conversations or to follow instructions.

A study published in the journal Brain Injury found that approximately 60% of individuals who had sustained a concussion reported difficulty with concentration or attention, which is a common symptom of distractibility.

Another study published in the journal Headache found that difficulty with concentration or attention was reported by approximately 70% of individuals with a concussion.

Nausea and vomiting

Some people with a concussion may experience nausea and vomiting. Nausea and vomiting are common symptoms of concussion, and may occur as a result of the brain being jarred or shaken inside the skull during the injury. Concussion-related nausea and vomiting may be accompanied by other symptoms, such as headache, dizziness, and fatigue.

Fatigue

A person with a concussion may feel tired or have trouble staying awake. Fatigue is a common symptom of concussion, and may occur as a result of the brain being jarred or shaken inside the skull during the injury. Concussion-related fatigue may manifest as a general feeling of tiredness or exhaustion, and may be accompanied by other symptoms, such as headache, dizziness, and difficulty with concentration and memory. Fatigue can range in severity from mild to severe. According to the Centers for Disease Control and Prevention (CDC), approximately 50% of people who sustain a concussion report experiencing fatigue as a symptom.

The severity and duration of fatigue after a concussion can vary depending on a number of factors, including the severity of the concussion, the patient's age and medical history, and other risk factors for fatigue. In general, fatigue after a concussion tends to be more severe and longer-lasting in those who have more severe or complicated concussions, and in those who have a history of fatigue or other underlying medical conditions that can cause fatigue.

Sensitivity to light and noise

A concussion can cause sensitivity to bright light or loud noises. Sensitivity to light and noise are common symptoms of concussion, and may occur as a result of the brain being jarred or shaken inside the skull during the injury. Concussion-related sensitivity to light and noise may manifest as discomfort or pain when exposed to bright lights or loud noises, and may be accompanied by other symptoms, such as headache, dizziness, and fatigue.

Sleep disturbance

A person with a concussion may have trouble falling asleep or may sleep more than usual. Concussion-related sleep impairment may manifest as difficulty falling asleep, staying asleep, or getting restful sleep, and may be accompanied by other symptoms, such as headache, dizziness, and fatigue.

Insomnia is a common sleep disorder that is characterised by difficulty falling or staying asleep, or by experiencing non-restorative sleep. Insomnia can be a symptom after a concussion, and can range in severity from mild to severe.

According to the Centers for Disease Control and Prevention (CDC), approximately 20-30% of people who sustain a concussion report experiencing insomnia as a symptom. Insomnia after a concussion may be caused by a variety of factors, including brain injury and changes in brain function, psychological factors such as stress, anxiety, and depression, and other medical conditions or medications that can affect sleep.

Mood changes

A concussion can cause mood changes, such as irritability, anxiety, or depression. Concussion-related mood changes may manifest as changes in emotional state, such as increased irritability, sadness, or anxiety, and may be accompanied by other symptoms, such as headache, dizziness, and fatigue.

Mood changes after a concussion can be caused by a range of factors, including physical fatigue, cognitive impairment, and emotional changes. Physical fatigue can make it difficult to regulate emotions and can lead to feelings of irritability or frustration. Cognitive impairment, such as difficulty with memory or concentration, can also contribute to mood changes. Emotional changes, such as depression or anxiety, can also be a result of a concussion. Emotional lability, also known as emotional instability, is a term used to describe a tendency to experience sudden, intense emotional responses that may be out of proportion to the situation. This can include changes in mood, such as sudden shifts from happiness to sadness, or sudden outbursts of anger or frustration.

Emotional lability can be a symptom of a concussion, which is a type of traumatic brain injury that occurs when the brain is jarred or shaken inside the skull. A concussion can cause damage to the brain and disrupt normal brain function, which can lead to changes in behaviour and mood.

Some research has suggested that mood changes after a concussion may be more common in older individuals or in those with more severe injuries.

A study published in the journal Brain Injury found that approximately 50% of individuals who had sustained a concussion reported mood changes, with about one-third reporting irritability and about one-quarter reporting anxiety or depression.

Another study published in the journal Headache found that mood changes were reported by approximately 25% of individuals with a concussion, with the most common changes being irritability (12%) and anxiety or depression (10%).

Lack of motivation

Lack of motivation can be a frustrating and distressing symptom of a concussion, as it can make it difficult to complete tasks or engage in activities that you normally enjoy. Lack of motivation can manifest in a variety of ways, such as difficulty initiating tasks or activities, difficulty completing tasks or activities, and a lack of interest in things that you normally enjoy. It can be a frustrating and distressing symptom, as it can make it difficult to engage in activities that you normally find rewarding or fulfilling.

Lack of motivation after a concussion can be caused by a range of factors, including physical fatigue, cognitive impairment, and emotional changes. Physical fatigue can make it difficult to find the energy to initiate or complete tasks. Cognitive impairment, such as difficulty with memory or concentration, can make it difficult to focus on tasks or to understand instructions. Emotional changes, such as depression or anxiety, can also contribute to lack of motivation.

Reduced libido

Concussion can sometimes cause a range of physical and cognitive symptoms, including changes in sexual function. Some individuals who have experienced a concussion may experience a reduced libido, or a decreased interest in sexual activity.

There are several potential mechanisms by which concussion could affect sexual function, including changes in hormone levels, fatigue, and changes in brain function. It is also possible that the physical or emotional stress of the injury, or the medications used to treat the injury, could contribute to changes in libido.

Symptoms of a concussion can range from mild to severe, and may not always be immediately apparent.

Hormonal abnormalities

It is possible for a concussion or mild traumatic brain injury (MTBI) to cause hormonal abnormalities. The brain is responsible for the production and regulation of many hormones in the body, and a concussion can disrupt these processes.

One hormone that may be affected by a concussion is cortisol, which is produced by the adrenal glands. Cortisol is involved in the body's stress response and helps regulate blood sugar levels, blood pressure, and immune function. A concussion may cause an abnormal increase in cortisol levels, which can lead to symptoms such as fatigue, anxiety, and difficulty concentrating.

Another hormone that may be affected by a concussion is thyroid hormone, which helps regulate metabolism. A concussion may cause an abnormal decrease in thyroid hormone levels, leading to symptoms such as fatigue, weight gain, and cold intolerance.

It is possible for a concussion to cause changes in a person's sense of smell. The sense of smell is controlled by the olfactory system, which is located in the brain. When the brain is injured, as can occur with a concussion, it can affect the normal functioning of the olfactory system and lead to changes in a person's sense of smell.

Some research has suggested that changes in sense of smell after a concussion may be more common in older individuals or in those with more severe injuries.

A study published in the journal Brain Injury found that approximately 35% of individuals who had sustained a concussion reported changes in their sense of smell. The changes reported included both an impaired sense of smell (anosmia) and a heightened sense of smell (hyperosmia).

Another study published in the journal Headache found that changes in sense of smell were reported by 37% of individuals with a concussion, with about one-third reporting an impaired sense of smell and the remainder reporting a heightened sense of smell.

It is possible for a concussion to cause changes in a person's sense of taste. The sense of taste is controlled by the gustatory system, which is located in the brain. When the brain is injured, as can occur with a concussion, it can affect the normal functioning of the gustatory system and lead to changes in a person's sense of taste.

A study published in the journal Brain Injury found that approximately 20% of individuals who had sustained a concussion reported changes in their sense of taste. The changes reported included both an impaired sense of taste (ageusia) and a heightened sense of taste (hypergeusia).

Another study published in the journal Headache found that changes in sense of taste were reported by 15% of individuals with a concussion, with about half reporting an impaired sense of taste and the remainder reporting a heightened sense of taste.

It is important to note that these studies may not be representative of the general population, as they included individuals who had sought medical attention for their concussion. It is also possible that some individuals with a concussion may not report changes in their sense of taste, or may not be aware of such changes.

Post-concussion personality change

Post-injury personality change (PIPC) refers to changes in a person's personality, behavior, and emotional functioning that occur after a traumatic brain injury (TBI). These changes can include changes in mood, impulsivity, aggression, irritability, and apathy. PIPC can have a significant impact on the individual's quality of life and ability to function in daily life.

The phenomenology of PIPC can vary widely among individuals, and can include changes in a person's emotional regulation, social interactions, and motivation. For example, some individuals may experience increased irritability and impulsivity, while others may experience apathy and a lack of motivation.

The nosology of PIPC is still being debated and researched, however, some researchers have proposed classifying PIPC as a subtype of TBI-related disorders, such as chronic traumatic encephalopathy (CTE) or post-traumatic neurodegeneration (PTND). Others have proposed classifying it as a unique disorder, separate from TBI-related disorders.

It's important to note that PIPC can be difficult to diagnose and treat, as it often co-occurs with other TBI-related disorders, such as depression, anxiety, and PTSD. A thorough assessment by a qualified healthcare professional, such as a neurologist or neuropsychologist, is crucial to identify and manage PIPC.

In summary, PIPC is a phenomenon characterized by changes in personality, behavior and emotional functioning that occur after TBI. The phenomenology and nosology of PIPC are still being researched and debated, but it's clear that PIPC can have a significant impact on the individual's quality of life, and a thorough assessment is crucial to identify and manage it.

Secondary anxiety disorder after a traumatic brain injury

Traumatic brain injury (TBI) can lead to a variety of mental health conditions, including secondary anxiety disorders. These disorders can occur as a result of the injury and can have a significant impact on the individual's quality of life.

Secondary anxiety disorders following TBI can include:

Generalized anxiety disorder (GAD)

GAD is characterized by excessive and unrealistic worry and anxiety about everyday events and activities.

Panic disorder

Panic disorder is characterized by recurrent and unexpected panic attacks, which are sudden episodes of intense fear or discomfort.

Post-traumatic stress disorder (PTSD)

PTSD is characterized by a persistent and excessive emotional response to a traumatic event, such as a TBI. Symptoms can include nightmares, flashbacks, and avoidance behaviors.

Social anxiety disorder

Social anxiety disorder is characterized by excessive and unrealistic fear of social situations and interactions.

Specific phobias

Specific phobias are characterized by excessive and unrealistic fear of specific objects or situations.

The prevalence of secondary anxiety disorders following TBI varies, but it is estimated that they can occur in up to 40% of individuals with TBI. These disorders can be difficult to diagnose and treat as they often co-occur with other TBI-related disorders, such as depression, and cognitive impairments.

A thorough assessment by a qualified healthcare professional, such as a neurologist, neuropsychologist or a mental health professional, is crucial to identify and manage these secondary anxiety disorders. A combination of pharmacological and psychological treatments, such as cognitive-behavioral therapy (CBT), have been found to be effective in treating secondary anxiety disorders following TBI.

Chapter 8

Post-concussion syndrome

Neurocognitive impairment due to mild TBI

Prolonged post-concussion syndrome (PCS) is a condition that can occur after a concussion, characterized by persistent symptoms such as headaches, dizziness, fatigue, and difficulty with memory and concentration. Post-concussion (post-concussive) syndrome (PCS) has been a much-debated topic. Muddled by conflicting findings regarding symptom duration, an absence of objective neurologic findings, inconsistencies in presentation, poorly understood aetiology, and significant methodologic problems in the literature, PCS remains controversial. Depending on the definition and the population examined, 29-90% of patients experience post-concussion symptoms shortly after the traumatic insult. Minor head injury and concussion are generally used interchangeably in the medical literature; however, it should be noted that the traditional definition of concussion precludes findings of intracranial haemorrhage on CT scan, whereas the definition minor head injury does not (though it does preclude the presence of a skull fracture). A minor head injury typically indicates a blow to the head with a brief period of loss of consciousness (LOC) or post-traumatic amnesia or disorientation. At presentation, the Glasgow Coma Scale (GCS) score ranges from 13-15. However, more recent literature suggests, and many clinicians concur, that a GCS score of 14 or 15 denotes an injury with a significantly less chance of intracranial injury on CT scan than a GCS score of 13. Although no universally accepted definition of post-concussion syndrome exists, most of the literature defines the syndrome as the development of at least 3 of the following symptoms: headache, dizziness, fatigue, irritability, impaired memory and concentration, insomnia, and lowered tolerance for noise and light. Confusion exists in the literature, with some authors defining it as symptoms of at least 3 months' duration, while others define it as symptoms appearing within the first week. The syndrome is loosely defined as symptom occurrence and persistence within several weeks after the initial insult. In defining persistent post-concussive syndrome (PPCS), most authors use greater than one month, and still others use 6 months or a year. However, it generally applies to ongoing chronic symptoms that continue past expected resolution. Based on the predominant clinical signs and symptoms, post-concussion syndrome is classified to the physiological subtype, with predominant symptoms these of exercise intolerance and global dysfunction of the brain and the autonomic nervous system, the Vestibulo-Ocular subtype with isolated dysfunction of vestibular or ocular systems, the Cervicogenic subtype, with isolated dysfunction of the cervical spine and/or the surrounding musculature and the mood-related subtype, with predominantly mood-related and cognitive symptoms with minimal physical examination findings.

The classification of PCS as "organic" or "functional" has been a topic of debate in the medical community.

"Organic" refers to a condition that has a specific, identifiable cause, such as a structural or physiological dysfunction. In the case of PCS, organic causes could include a brain injury or changes in brain chemistry.

"Functional" refers to a condition that does not have a specific, identifiable cause, but is thought to be related to psychological or emotional factors, such as anxiety or depression.

Some experts believe that PCS is primarily an organic condition, caused by ongoing brain injury or changes in brain chemistry. Others believe that it is primarily a functional condition, caused by psychological or emotional factors.

It's important to note that the classification of PCS as organic or functional is not mutually exclusive and the two may overlap, as there are different factors that contribute to the development and persistence of PCS.

In most cases, PCS is thought to be multifactorial in nature, meaning that it is likely caused by a combination of organic and functional factors. It is important to evaluate and treat the patient as a whole, considering all the contributing factors in the development of PCS, and not just the organic causes.

Chapter 9

Diagnostic tools and techniques

Diagnosing mTBI and PCS

There are several diagnostic tools and techniques that can be used to diagnose a concussion. These may include:

Physical examination

A doctor will conduct a physical examination to assess the person's symptoms and any physical signs of a concussion, such as bruising or swelling.

Neurological examination

A neurological examination involves tests of the person's mental status, such as memory and cognitive function, as well as tests of their reflexes, muscle strength, and coordination.

Neuroimaging

Neuroimaging techniques, such as CT (computed tomography) scans or MRIs (magnetic resonance imaging), can be used to visualize the brain and look for signs of injury or bleeding.

Balance and coordination tests

Balance and coordination tests, such as the Balance Error Scoring System (BESS) or the Sport Concussion Assessment Tool (SCAT), can be used to assess the person's balance and coordination and determine the severity of their concussion.

Symptom checklists

Symptom checklists, such as the Concussion Symptom Inventory (CSI) or the Post-Concussion Symptom Scale (PCSS), can be used to assess the person's symptoms and monitor their recovery over time.

Diagnosing a concussion requires a combination of these tools and techniques, as well as a thorough medical history and evaluation of the person's symptoms. It is important to seek medical attention if you or someone you know experiences a concussion, as early diagnosis and treatment can help to prevent long-term complications and ensure a full recovery.

The ImPact test

The impact test is a type of cognitive assessment tool that is often used to evaluate the severity of concussion or other types of traumatic brain injury (TBI). It is also known as the Immediate Post-Concussion Assessment and Cognitive Testing (ImPACT) test.

The ImPACT test consists of a series of computerized tasks that measure various cognitive functions, such as attention, memory, processing speed, and reaction time. It also includes a symptom checklist that asks the individual to report any symptoms they are experiencing, such as headache, dizziness, or fatigue.

The ImPACT test is usually administered on a computer and takes about 20-30 minutes to complete. It is typically administered twice: once shortly after the injury (within 48-72 hours) and again a few days later. The results of the test are then compared to a baseline test that was taken before the injury, and any changes in performance are used to evaluate the severity of the concussion and guide treatment decisions.

It is important to note that the ImPACT test is not a standalone diagnostic tool and should not be used as the sole basis for determining whether or not an individual has sustained a concussion. It is intended to be used as part of a comprehensive evaluation by a healthcare provider. Other factors, such as the individual's symptoms, physical examination, and imaging studies, should also be taken into consideration when evaluating a potential concussion.

Post concussion symptoms scale

Post-concussion syndrome (PCS) is a set of symptoms that can occur after a concussion or other traumatic brain injury (TBI). These symptoms can include physical, cognitive, and emotional symptoms, and they can vary widely in severity and duration.

There are several different scales that have been developed to assess the severity of PCS and track changes over time. One example is the Post-Concussion Symptom Inventory (PCSI), which is a self-report questionnaire that measures the severity of a range of physical, cognitive, and emotional symptoms commonly experienced after a concussion. The PCSI includes 22 symptom items and asks the individual to rate the severity of each symptom on a scale of 0 (not at all) to 6 (extremely).

Another example is the Rivermead Post-Concussion Symptoms Questionnaire (RPQ), which is also a self-report questionnaire that measures the severity of a range of physical, cognitive, and emotional symptoms. The RPQ includes 16 symptom items and asks the individual to rate the severity of each symptom on a scale of 0 (not at all) to 4 (extremely).

These scales can be used to help identify the presence and severity of PCS, as well as to track changes in symptoms over time. They can be helpful in guiding treatment decisions and determining the need for further evaluation or referral to a specialist. It is important to note that these scales are not diagnostic tools and should be used in conjunction with a comprehensive evaluation by a healthcare provider.

Chapter 10

Diagnostic criteria for PCS

DSM V and ICD-10

DSM V criteria

Post-concussion syndrome (PCS) is not a specific diagnosis listed in the Diagnostic and Statistical Manual of Mental Disorders (DSM-5), which is the manual used by mental health professionals in the United States to diagnose mental health conditions. However, the DSM-5 does include a category called "Other specified neurocognitive disorder" (OSND) which may be used to diagnose individuals with symptoms that may be consistent with PCS.

To diagnose OSND, the DSM-5 requires that the individual has experienced a recent neurological insult, such as a concussion or brain injury, and is experiencing cognitive symptoms that are not better explained by another mental disorder or medical condition. The DSM-5 lists the following as potential symptoms of OSND:

- Impaired attention and concentration
- Memory problems
- Slowed thinking and processing speed
- Difficulty with executive functioning (e.g., planning and organization)
- Disorientation or confusion
- Mood changes (e.g., irritability, anxiety, or depression)

To diagnose OSND, these symptoms must be present for at least four weeks and must be severe enough to interfere with the individual's daily functioning. It is important to note that the DSM-5 does not specify a specific set of criteria for diagnosing PCS, as it is not a specific diagnosis. Rather, it is a group of symptoms that may be experienced after a concussion or brain injury.

ICD-10 criteria

According to the International Classification of Diseases, 10th edition (ICD-10), the criteria for post-concussion syndrome (PCS) are as follows:

A history of a concussion, defined as a transient alteration of mental status after a blow to the head or body, or from a rapid acceleration or deceleration of the head.

Persistent symptoms that occur after the concussion, including at least one of the following:

- Headache
- Dizziness
- Fatigue
- Irritability
- Anxiety
- Depression

The symptoms must not be due to another medical condition, and must not be better explained by another disorder.

It is important to note that the diagnosis of PCS is based on the presence of persistent symptoms after a concussion, and does not require a specific number or severity of symptoms. The diagnosis of PCS is typically made by a healthcare provider based on a thorough evaluation of the patient's history, physical examination, and other relevant tests and assessments.

Chapter 11

Biomarkers

Fluid and Imaging Biomarkers for PCS

Biomarkers are biological molecules or characteristics that can be measured and used as indicators of a particular biological process or disease state. Biomarkers can be found in a variety of body fluids and tissues, including blood, urine, and cerebrospinal fluid (CSF).

In the context of brain injuries, biomarkers can be used to help diagnose and monitor the severity of injury, as well as to predict the likelihood of long-term recovery or complications. Some examples of biomarkers that have been studied in the context of brain injuries include:

Neuronal injury biomarkers

These biomarkers are released by damaged neurons and can be used to indicate the extent of neuronal injury. Examples include neuron-specific enolase (NSE) and tau protein.

Inflammatory biomarkers

These biomarkers are released by immune cells in response to injury or inflammation and can be used to measure the level of inflammation in the brain. Examples include interleukin-6 (IL-6) and tumor necrosis factor-alpha (TNF-alpha).

Oxidative stress biomarkers

These biomarkers are produced as a result of oxidative stress, which is an imbalance between the production of reactive oxygen species (ROS) and the ability of the body to neutralize them. ROS can cause damage to cells and tissues, and high levels of oxidative stress have been linked to poor outcomes in brain injury. Examples of oxidative stress biomarkers include malondialdehyde (MDA) and 8-hydroxy-2'-deoxyguanosine (8-OHdG).

It is important to note that while biomarkers can be useful tools for diagnosing and monitoring brain injuries, they are not the only factors that determine the severity of injury or the likelihood of recovery. Other factors, such as the type and location of the injury, the age of the individual, and the presence of other medical conditions, can also influence outcomes.

CT scan

A CT scan, also known as a computed tomography (CT) scan or a computed axial tomography (CAT) scan, is a type of medical imaging test that uses X-rays and a computer to create detailed images of the inside of the body. CT scans are often used to diagnose and monitor a wide range of medical conditions, including injuries to the head and brain.

During a CT scan, the individual lies on a table that is moved through a circular opening in a large machine. The machine rotates around the head, taking a series of detailed X-ray images as it goes. These images are then combined using a computer to create detailed cross-sectional images of the brain.

CT scans are fast, painless, and non-invasive, and they do not require any special preparation. They are typically performed in a hospital or outpatient imaging center, and the entire process takes about 30 minutes.

CT scans are generally very safe, although they do expose the individual to a small amount of ionizing radiation. In most cases, the benefits of the scan outweigh the risks of radiation exposure. However, pregnant women and children may be more sensitive to radiation and may require alternative imaging tests.

CT scans are often used to evaluate head injuries, including concussions, skull fractures, and brain bleeds. They can also be used to diagnose other medical conditions that affect the brain, such as brain tumors, aneurysms, and stroke. CT scans are typically more accurate than other types of imaging tests, such as X-rays, at detecting abnormalities in the brain, but they may not be as detailed as more specialized imaging tests, such as MRI.

MRI scan

Magnetic resonance imaging (MRI) is a medical imaging technique that uses a strong magnetic field and radio waves to create detailed images of the inside of the body. MRI scans are often used to diagnose and monitor a wide range of medical conditions, including injuries to the head and brain.

During an MRI scan, the individual lies on a table that is moved into a large, cylindrical machine called an MRI scanner. The scanner produces a strong magnetic field and radio waves, which are used to create detailed images of the brain and other organs. The scan typically takes 30-60 minutes to complete.

MRI scans are non-invasive, painless, and do not expose the individual to ionizing radiation, making them a safe and widely used imaging technique. However, MRI scanners can be loud and may be uncomfortable for some individuals, especially those who are claustrophobic or have a fear of enclosed spaces.

MRI scans can produce detailed images of the brain and can be used to evaluate a wide range of conditions, including brain injuries, brain tumours, aneurysms, and strokes. They are often more detailed than other types of imaging tests, such as CT scans, and can provide additional information about the structure and function of the brain.

MRI scans can be particularly useful for evaluating concussion, also known as mild traumatic brain injury (mTBI), because they can provide detailed images of the brain and can help to identify abnormalities that may not be visible on other types of imaging tests, such as CT scans. MRI scans can also be used to evaluate the extent of brain tissue damage and the presence of other conditions, such as brain bleeds or swelling, that may be associated with concussion.

It is important to note that MRI scans may not be suitable for all individuals, particularly those with certain types of implanted medical devices, such as pacemakers or certain types of cochlear implants. In these cases, alternative imaging tests, such as CT scans, may be used.

However, it is important to note that MRI scans are not always necessary for the diagnosis and management of concussion. In many cases, a concussion can be diagnosed based on the individual's symptoms, physical examination, and other imaging tests, such as CT scans. MRI scans may be reserved for cases where the individual is experiencing persistent or severe symptoms, or when there are other concerns that need to be addressed.

EEG

An electroencephalogram (EEG) is a test that measures the electrical activity of the brain. It is often used to diagnose and monitor conditions that affect the brain, such as epilepsy, brain tumors, and head injuries, including concussion.

During an EEG test, a healthcare provider places small electrodes on the individual's scalp. These electrodes are connected to a machine that records the brain's electrical activity. The test typically takes 20-30 minutes to complete and is painless.

EEG tests can be helpful in the evaluation of concussion because they can provide information about the brain's electrical activity and can help to identify any abnormal activity that may be present. For example, an EEG test may show changes in brain activity that are consistent with concussion, such as slowing of brain waves or abnormal bursts of activity.

EEG tests are generally safe and non-invasive, and they do not expose the individual to ionizing radiation. However, they may not be suitable for all individuals, particularly those with certain types of implanted medical devices, such as pacemakers. In these cases, alternative testing methods may be used.

It is important to note that EEG tests are not a standalone diagnostic tool and should be used in conjunction with a comprehensive evaluation by a healthcare provider. Other factors, such as the individual's symptoms, medical history, and the specific circumstances of the injury, should also be taken into consideration when evaluating and managing a concussion.

Chapter 12

Treatment and Recovery

Overview of treatment options

Treatment for a concussion will depend on the severity of the injury and the individual's symptoms. In most cases, the best treatment for a concussion is rest and time. This may involve taking a break from physical activity, including sports and other high-energy activities, and avoiding tasks that require mental effort, such as reading or watching television. It is also important to get plenty of sleep and avoid substances that can worsen concussion symptoms, such as alcohol and caffeine.

Over-the-counter pain medications, such as acetaminophen/paracetamol or ibuprofen, can be used to manage headache and other pain symptoms. Some people may also benefit from physical therapy or other rehabilitation techniques to help with balance and coordination. Taking over the counter pain medication should be avoided because of the risk of rebound headaches. Seeking medical assistance is always critical.

In more severe cases, a concussion may require more intensive treatment, such as hospitalization or surgery. This may be necessary if the person has lost consciousness, has severe symptoms, or has a brain bleed or other serious brain injury.

It is important to follow the recommended treatment plan and seek medical attention if symptoms worsen or do not improve. Early diagnosis and treatment can help to prevent long-term complications and ensure a full recovery.

Importance of proper management and care to support recovery

Proper management and care are important to support recovery from a concussion. This may include:

Rest and time

Taking a break from physical and mental activity, including sports and other high-energy activities, and getting plenty of sleep can help to support recovery from a concussion.

Medication

Over-the-counter pain medications, such as acetaminophen or ibuprofen, can be used to manage headache and other pain symptoms.

Rehabilitation

Physical therapy or other rehabilitation techniques can help with balance and coordination and support recovery from a concussion.

Follow-up care

It is important to follow up with a healthcare provider after experiencing a concussion to ensure that symptoms are improving and to monitor for any long-term complications.

Proper management and care can help to prevent long-term complications and ensure a full recovery from a concussion. If you or someone you know has experienced a concussion, it is important to seek medical attention and follow the recommended treatment plan.

Non pharmaceutical treatments

Non pharmaceutical treatments for post concussion headaches

Non-pharmacological treatments for post-concussion headaches may include the following:

Cognitive behavioral therapy (CBT)

CBT is a type of therapy that aims to identify and change negative thought patterns and behaviors that contribute to headaches. It may include techniques such as relaxation training and stress management.

Exercise

Regular physical activity may help reduce the frequency and severity of headaches by promoting relaxation and reducing stress. It is important to avoid vigorous exercise if you are experiencing a headache, as it may exacerbate the pain.

Chiropractic care

Chiropractic care involves the use of manual adjustments to the spine and other joints to improve function and alleviate pain. Some studies have shown that chiropractic care may be effective in reducing the frequency and severity of headaches.

Acupuncture

Acupuncture is a form of traditional Chinese medicine that involves the insertion of thin needles into specific points on the body to promote healing and relieve pain. Some studies have shown that acupuncture may be effective in reducing the frequency and severity of headaches.

Massage therapy

Massage therapy involves the manipulation of the muscles and tissues to promote relaxation and alleviate pain. It may be effective in reducing the frequency and severity of headaches.

It is important to note that non-pharmacological treatments for post-concussion headaches may not be suitable for everyone, and may not be effective in all cases. If you are experiencing headaches and are considering non-pharmacological treatments, it is important to discuss your options with a healthcare provider. They will be able to provide more information and advice based on your specific situation.

Non pharmaceutical treatments for memory impairment after concussion

Non-pharmacological treatments for memory impairment after a concussion may include the following:

Cognitive rehabilitation therapy

This type of therapy involves structured activities and exercises designed to improve cognitive function, including memory. It may involve tasks such as memory drills, problem-solving activities, and language exercises. CBT aims to identify and change negative thought patterns and behaviors that contribute to cognitive impairments. It may include techniques such as relaxation training and stress management.

Exercise

Regular physical activity may help improve cognitive function, including memory, by promoting brain health and increasing blood flow to the brain.

Nutrition

A healthy diet rich in fruits, vegetables, and omega-3 fatty acids may help support brain health and improve cognitive function.

Sleep

Adequate sleep is important for brain health and cognitive function. Establishing a consistent sleep schedule and practicing good sleep hygiene may help improve memory and cognitive function.

It is important to note that non-pharmacological treatments for memory impairment after a concussion may not be suitable for everyone, and may not be effective in all cases. If you are experiencing memory impairment and are considering non-pharmacological treatments, it is important to discuss your options with a healthcare provider. They will be able to provide more information and advice based on your specific situation.

Non pharmaceutical treatments for post concussion depression

Non-pharmacological treatments for post-concussion depression may include the following:

Cognitive behavioral therapy (CBT)

CBT is a type of therapy that aims to identify and change negative thought patterns and behaviors that contribute to depression. It may involve techniques such as relaxation training, stress management, and problem-solving skills.

Exercise

Regular physical activity may help reduce the symptoms of depression by promoting relaxation, reducing stress, and increasing the production of feel-good chemicals in the brain.

Light therapy: Light therapy involves exposure to bright light, which may help improve mood and reduce the symptoms of depression.

Social support

Spending time with friends and loved ones and participating in activities that you enjoy may help improve mood and reduce the symptoms of depression.

Self-care

Engaging in activities such as meditation, yoga, or journaling may help reduce stress and improve mood.

It is important to note that non-pharmacological treatments for post-concussion depression may not be suitable for everyone, and may not be effective in all cases. If you are experiencing depression and are considering non-pharmacological treatments, it is important to discuss your options with a healthcare provider. They will be able to provide more information and advice based on your specific situation.

Non pharmaceutical treatments for post concussion dizziness

Non-pharmacological treatments for post-concussion dizziness may include the following:

Vestibular rehabilitation therapy

This type of therapy involves exercises and activities designed to improve balance and coordination and reduce dizziness. It may include balance training, eye movement exercises, and head and neck exercises.

Exercise

Regular physical activity may help improve balance and reduce dizziness by promoting relaxation and increasing blood flow to the brain.

Relaxation techniques

Techniques such as deep breathing, progressive muscle relaxation, and meditation may help reduce dizziness by promoting relaxation and reducing stress.

Nutrition

A healthy diet rich in fruits, vegetables, and omega-3 fatty acids may help support overall health and reduce dizziness.

Sleep

Adequate sleep is important for overall health and well-being, and may help reduce dizziness. Establishing a consistent sleep schedule and practicing good sleep hygiene may help improve dizziness.

It is important to note that non-pharmacological treatments for post-concussion dizziness may not be suitable for everyone, and may not be effective in all cases. If you are experiencing dizziness and are considering non-pharmacological treatments, it is important to discuss your options with a healthcare provider. They will be able to provide more information and advice based on your specific situation.

Non pharmaceutical treatments for post concussion behavioural changes

Non-pharmacological treatments for post-concussion behavioral changes may include the following:

Cognitive behavioral therapy (CBT)

CBT is a type of therapy that aims to identify and change negative thought patterns and behaviors that contribute to behavioral changes. It may involve techniques such as relaxation training, stress management, and problem-solving skills.

Exercise

Regular physical activity may help improve mood and reduce stress, which may in turn help improve behavioral changes.

Nutrition

A healthy diet rich in fruits, vegetables, and omega-3 fatty acids may help support overall health and improve mood.

Sleep

Adequate sleep is important for overall health and well-being, and may help improve behavioral changes. Establishing a consistent sleep schedule and practicing good sleep hygiene may help improve behavioral changes.

Social support

Spending time with friends and loved ones and participating in activities that you enjoy may help improve mood and reduce stress, which may in turn help improve behavioral changes.

It is important to note that non-pharmacological treatments for post-concussion behavioral changes may not be suitable for everyone, and may not be effective in all cases. If you are experiencing behavioral changes and are considering non-pharmacological treatments, it is important to discuss your options with a healthcare provider. They will be able to provide more information and advice based on your specific situation.

Non pharmaceutical treatments for post concussion reduced libido

Non-pharmacological treatments for post-concussion reduced libido may include the following:

Cognitive behavioral therapy (CBT)

CBT is a type of therapy that aims to identify and change negative thought patterns and behaviors that contribute to reduced libido. It may involve techniques such as relaxation training and stress management.

Exercise

Regular physical activity may help improve libido by promoting relaxation and reducing stress.

Nutrition

A healthy diet rich in fruits, vegetables, and omega-3 fatty acids may help support overall health and improve libido.

Sleep

Adequate sleep is important for overall health and well-being, and may help improve libido. Establishing a consistent sleep schedule and practicing good sleep hygiene may help improve libido.

Communication

Open and honest communication with a partner about sexual desires and concerns may help improve libido and intimacy.

It is important to note that non-pharmacological treatments for post-concussion reduced libido may not be suitable for everyone, and may not be effective in all cases. If you are experiencing reduced libido and are considering non-pharmacological treatments, it is important to discuss your options with a healthcare provider. They will be able to provide more information and advice based on your specific situation.

Non pharmaceutical treatments of insomnia after concussion

Non-pharmacological approaches for managing sleep abnormalities, such as insomnia, may include the following:

Cognitive behavioral therapy for insomnia (CBT-I)

CBT-I is a type of therapy that aims to identify and change negative thought patterns and behaviors that contribute to insomnia. CBT-I may include techniques such as sleep restriction, stimulus control, and relaxation training.

Lifestyle changes

Making certain changes to your daily routine and habits may help improve your sleep quality. These may include setting a consistent bedtime and wake-up time, avoiding caffeine and alcohol before bedtime, and creating a relaxing bedtime routine.

Relaxation techniques

Techniques such as deep breathing, progressive muscle relaxation, and visualization can help reduce stress and promote relaxation, which may improve sleep quality.

Exercise

Regular physical activity may help improve sleep quality by promoting relaxation and reducing stress. It is important to avoid vigorous exercise close to bedtime, as it may stimulate the body and make it harder to fall asleep.

Sleep hygiene

Practicing good sleep hygiene, such as keeping a cool and comfortable sleep environment, avoiding screens before bedtime, and reducing exposure to noise and light, may help improve sleep quality.

It is important to note that non-pharmacological approaches for managing sleep abnormalities may not be suitable for everyone, and may not be effective in all cases. If you are experiencing sleep abnormalities and are considering non-pharmacological approaches, it is important to discuss your options with a healthcare provider. They will be able to provide more information and advice based on your specific situation.

Coping with Emotional and Psychological Effects

Concussions can have emotional and psychological effects, such as mood changes, difficulty with memory and concentration, and changes in personality. Coping with these effects can be challenging, but there are strategies that can help. Some strategies for coping with the emotional and psychological effects of a concussion include:

Seek support

It can be helpful to seek support from friends, family, or a support group to help cope with the emotional and psychological effects of a concussion. Talking to others who have experienced similar challenges can be a valuable source of support and understanding.

Talk to a therapist

A therapist or other mental health professional can provide specialized support and guidance for coping with the emotional and psychological effects of a concussion. They can help identify coping strategies and provide a safe space to talk about and process feelings.

Practice relaxation techniques

Relaxation techniques such as deep breathing, meditation, or progressive muscle relaxation can help manage stress and improve mood.

Engage in activities that are enjoyable

Engaging in activities that are enjoyable and bring a sense of accomplishment can help improve mood and provide a sense of purpose. This may include hobbies, social activities, or volunteering.

Seek medical attention

If the emotional and psychological effects of a concussion are severe or interfere with daily life, it may be necessary to seek medical attention. A healthcare provider can assess the situation and recommend treatment options such as medication or therapy.

Overall, it is important to seek support and find coping strategies that work for you to help manage the emotional and psychological effects of a concussion. It is also important to seek medical attention if needed.

Chapter 13

Living with a concussion

Copying with symptoms and needs

Living with a concussion can be challenging and overwhelming, as it can cause a range of physical, emotional, and cognitive symptoms that can disrupt daily life. Some common challenges of living with a concussion include:

Physical symptoms

Concussions can cause a wide range of physical symptoms, such as headaches, dizziness, fatigue, and difficulty with balance and coordination. These symptoms can be difficult to manage and can disrupt activities such as work, school, and exercise.

Emotional and psychological effects

Concussions can also have emotional and psychological effects, such as mood changes, difficulty with memory and concentration, and changes in personality. These effects can be distressing and can make it difficult to engage in activities that were previously enjoyable.

Disruption of daily life

Concussions can disrupt daily routines and activities, as people may need to take time off work or school, limit their physical activity, and make other changes in order to recover. This can be difficult to adjust to and can cause stress and frustration.

Difficulty seeking help

It can be difficult for people with concussions to identify and communicate their symptoms, which can make it challenging to seek help and get the support they need. Some people may also feel ashamed or embarrassed about their concussion and may be reluctant to seek help.

Long-term effects

In some cases, concussions can have long-term effects that persist even after the initial injury has healed. These effects can be difficult to manage and may require ongoing medical care and support.

The importance of seeking medical attention

Seeking medical attention and following treatment recommendations is crucial for people with concussions. This is because concussions are serious injuries that can have significant long-term consequences if not properly treated. Some reasons why seeking medical attention and following treatment recommendations is important include:

Concussions can have serious long-term effects

Without proper treatment, concussions can have long-term effects on brain function, including problems with memory, concentration, and mood. Seeking medical attention and following treatment recommendations can help prevent these long-term effects.

Concussions can lead to more serious injuries

If a person with a concussion continues to engage in activities that could cause further injury, they may be at risk of more serious injuries such as a brain bleed or brain swelling. Seeking medical attention and following treatment recommendations can help prevent these complications.

Concussions can interfere with daily life Concussions can cause symptoms such as headaches, dizziness, and fatigue that can disrupt daily life and make it difficult to engage in work, school, and other activities. Seeking medical attention and following treatment recommendations can help alleviate these symptoms and allow people to return to their daily lives more quickly.

Treatment can help speed recovery

Following treatment recommendations, such as taking medications as prescribed and avoiding activities that could cause further injury, can help speed recovery and reduce the risk of long-term consequences.

Overall, seeking medical attention and following treatment recommendations is essential for people with concussions in order to ensure proper care and prevent long-term consequences.

Strategies to manage symptoms

There are a number of strategies that people with concussions can use to manage common symptoms such as headaches, dizziness, and fatigue. Some of these strategies include:

Managing headaches: To manage headaches, people with concussions may find it helpful to:

- Take over-the-counter pain medication as directed
- Use a cold or warm compress to help alleviate pain
- Avoid activities that could exacerbate the headache, such as strenuous physical activity or staring at screens for long periods of time
- Practice relaxation techniques such as deep breathing or meditation

Managing dizziness

To manage dizziness, people with concussions may find it helpful to:

- Avoid sudden movements or changes in position
- Take breaks and rest often
- Avoid bright lights or loud noises
- Use a cane or other assistive device if needed

Managing fatigue

To manage fatigue, people with concussions may find it helpful to:

- Get plenty of rest, including taking naps as needed
- Avoid strenuous physical activity or other activities that could cause fatigue
- Pace themselves and take breaks often
- Eat a healthy diet and stay hydrated

It is important to note that everyone is different and may experience different symptoms and have different ways of managing them. It is important to consult with a healthcare professional for specific recommendations on how to manage symptoms.

Tips for getting enough rest and managing stress

Getting enough rest and managing stress are important for people with concussions as they can help alleviate symptoms and speed recovery. Some tips for getting enough rest and managing stress include:

Get plenty of sleep

Getting enough sleep is important for people with concussions, as it can help the brain heal and improve symptoms such as fatigue and difficulty concentrating. It is generally recommended that people with concussions aim for at least 7-9 hours of sleep per night.

Create a relaxing sleep environment Creating a comfortable and relaxing sleep environment can help improve sleep quality. This may include keeping the bedroom cool, dark, and quiet, using a comfortable mattress and pillows, and avoiding screens before bed.

Take naps as needed

If fatigue is a problem, taking short naps during the day can help alleviate fatigue and improve symptoms. It is important to avoid napping for too long, as this can disrupt sleep patterns.

Manage stress

Stress can worsen concussion symptoms and interfere with recovery. Strategies for managing stress include:

- Practice relaxation techniques such as deep breathing or meditation
- Engage in activities that are relaxing, such as reading, listening to music, or going for a walk

- Talk to a therapist or other mental health professional
- Avoid activities that are overly stimulating or stressful
- Seek support from friends, family, or a support group

It is important to note that everyone is different and may have different strategies for getting enough rest and managing stress. It is important to consult with a healthcare professional for specific recommendations on how to manage these issues.

Chapter 14

Returning to Work and Other Activities

Return to work

Returning to work and other activities after a concussion can be a challenging process, as it is important to balance the need for rest and recovery with the desire to get back to normal activities. Here are some tips for returning to work and other activities after a concussion:

Take things slowly

It is important to take things slowly and not try to do too much too soon after a concussion. This may mean starting with small amounts of activity and gradually increasing as symptoms improve.

Communicate with your employer or school

It is important to communicate with your employer or school about your concussion and any accommodations you may need in order to return to work or school safely. This may include adjustments to your work schedule, temporary reassignment to less demanding tasks, or other accommodations.

Gradually return to activities

Gradually returning to activities can help prevent a setback in recovery. This may mean starting with less demanding activities and gradually increasing intensity and duration as symptoms improve.

Listen to your body

It is important to listen to your body and pay attention to any symptoms that may indicate that you are doing too much. If you experience an increase in symptoms such as headache, dizziness, or fatigue, it may be necessary to reduce activity or rest.

Overall, it is important to take a gradual and careful approach to returning to work and other activities after a concussion, as this can help ensure a smooth and successful recovery. It is also important to consult with a healthcare professional for specific recommendations on how to return to work and other activities safely.

The importance of taking things slowly and not overdoing it

It is important to take things slowly and not overdo it after a concussion, as this can help ensure a smooth and successful recovery. Here are some reasons why taking things slowly and not overdoing it is important:

Rest is crucial for recovery

Rest is an important part of the recovery process after a concussion, as it gives the brain time to heal. Engaging in too much activity too soon can interfere with this process and delay recovery.

Overdoing it can worsen symptoms Engaging in too much activity too soon can worsen symptoms such as headache, dizziness, and fatigue, which can set back recovery. It is important to listen to your body and pay attention to any symptoms that may indicate that you are doing too much.

Overdoing it can increase the risk of further injury

If a person with a concussion continues to engage in activities that could cause further injury, they may be at risk of more serious injuries such as a brain bleed or brain swelling. Taking things slowly and not overdoing it can help reduce this risk.

Overall, taking things slowly and not overdoing it is important for people with concussions in order to ensure a smooth and successful recovery and prevent further injury. It is important to consult with a healthcare professional for specific recommendations on how to manage activity levels after a concussion.

Tips for communicating with your employer or school about your concussion

It is important to communicate with your employer or school about your concussion and any accommodations you may need in order to return to work or school safely. Here are some tips for communicating with your employer or school about your concussion:

Be proactive

It is important to be proactive in communicating with your employer or school about your concussion and any accommodations you may need. This may include letting them know about any symptoms you are experiencing and any restrictions on your activity level.

Follow your treatment plan

Following your treatment plan and keeping your healthcare provider informed about your progress can help demonstrate your commitment to your recovery and your readiness to return to work or school.

Understand your rights

It is important to understand your rights under laws such as the Americans with Disabilities Act (ADA) and the Family and Medical Leave Act (FMLA), which may provide protections and accommodations for people with disabilities, including concussions.

Seek help if needed

If you are having difficulty communicating with your employer or school about your concussion, it may be helpful to seek the assistance of a healthcare provider, a disability rights advocate, or an attorney.

Overall, effective communication with your employer or school about your concussion and any accommodations you may need can help ensure a smooth and successful return to work or school. It is important to be proactive and seek help if needed in order to get the support you need.

Chapter 15

Video games and Neurofeedback in concussion rehabilitation

The role of video games and neurofeedback

There is some evidence that video games can be used as a tool for concussion rehabilitation. Concussions are injuries to the brain that can cause a range of symptoms, including headache, dizziness, difficulty concentrating, and memory problems. Rehabilitation after a concussion often involves rest and gradually returning to normal activities, as well as exercises to help improve cognitive function.

One way that video games may be used in concussion rehabilitation is through the use of "brain games" or other cognitive training programs. These types of games are designed to improve brain function and are often used in rehabilitation settings to help patients improve their memory, attention, and other cognitive skills. Some research has suggested that playing these types of games may be beneficial for concussion recovery, although more research is needed to fully understand their effectiveness.

It is important to note that video games should not be used as a replacement for medical treatment or rehabilitation following a concussion. If you or someone you know has sustained a concussion, it is important to follow the recommended treatment plan provided by a healthcare provider.

Neurofeedback, also known as EEG biofeedback, is a type of therapy that involves using feedback from an individual's brain waves to help them learn to control their brain activity. Neurofeedback has been studied as a potential treatment for a variety of conditions, including concussion, also known as mild traumatic brain injury (mTBI).

In the context of concussion treatment, neurofeedback may be used to help individuals with persistent symptoms, such as headaches, fatigue, and difficulty with concentration and memory. The therapy involves using sensors to measure brain activity and providing the individual with feedback about their brain waves, typically in the form of a visual or auditory signal. The individual is then asked to try to change their brain activity in a specific way, such as by relaxing or focusing, in order to improve their symptoms.

There is some evidence to suggest that neurofeedback may be effective in reducing symptoms and improving function in individuals with concussion. However, the research on neurofeedback for concussion treatment is limited and more research is needed to fully understand its effectiveness.

It is important to note that neurofeedback is not a standalone treatment for concussion and should be used in conjunction with a comprehensive treatment plan that may include other therapies, such as physical therapy, occupational therapy, and medication management. It is also important to speak with a healthcare provider about the potential risks and benefits of neurofeedback and other treatment options.

Chapter 16

Exercise and diet

The role of exercise and diet

Incorporating exercise into the rehabilitation process following a mild traumatic brain injury (MTBI), commonly known as a concussion, can significantly contribute to a patient's recovery. Nonetheless, it is crucial to approach physical activity with caution and under the guidance of a healthcare professional to ensure that the exercise regimen aligns with the individual's recovery phase and symptomatology.

Understanding the Role of Exercise Post-Concussion

After experiencing an MTBI, individuals often face symptoms like headaches, fatigue, dizziness, and difficulties with concentration and memory. These symptoms can hinder one's capacity to engage in physical activities at their pre-injury level. The key to reintroducing exercise after a concussion lies in a carefully monitored, stepwise approach that respects the body's signals and the brain's need for recovery.

Gradual Resumption of Physical Activity

Initiating exercise post-concussion should be a gradual process, starting with low-intensity activities that do not provoke symptoms. The gradual increase in the intensity and duration of exercise should only proceed as tolerated, without exacerbating symptoms. It's imperative for individuals to stay attuned to their body's responses and to cease exercising immediately should any symptoms worsen during or after physical activity.

Recommended Types of Exercise After MTBI

Cardiovascular Exercise: Engaging in aerobic activities can enhance cardiovascular health, aid in stress management, and uplift mood, which is particularly beneficial during the recovery from a concussion. Activities such as gentle walking, stationary cycling, and swimming are ideal, as they are less likely to jostle the head and exacerbate symptoms.

Strength Training

Gradually incorporating strength training exercises can bolster muscle strength and improve overall balance. This is crucial for preventing falls, which could potentially worsen the condition or lead to additional injuries. However, heavy lifting should be approached with caution, and any activity that strains the neck or head should be avoided or closely monitored.

Balance Exercises

Balance and coordination may be compromised following an MTBI. Exercises designed to enhance these abilities are essential and can include simple practices such as standing on one leg, using a balance board, or engaging in tai chi. These activities help retrain the brain and improve proprioception, which is often affected after a concussion.

Weight Lifting Programs Post-Concussion

When considering weight lifting post-concussion, it's critical to have a tailored program designed by a healthcare professional familiar with your case. The program's initiation should be predicated on the severity of the concussion and any persisting symptoms. It's generally advisable to start with light weights and high repetitions, avoiding any form of strain or pressure that could induce headaches or worsen neurological symptoms.

Conclusion

Exercise, when appropriately timed and progressively scaled, can play a significant role in the recovery from a concussion. By adhering to medical advice and listening to their bodies, individuals can navigate their path to recovery with an exercise regimen that supports their healing process. Always remember, the primary goal post-concussion is to recover fully, and exercise should be a part of this process, not a hindrance.

Cardio exercise

Integrating exercise into the recovery plan for individuals who have experienced a mild traumatic brain injury (MTBI) or are dealing with post-concussion syndrome (PCS) is a nuanced process that requires careful consideration and professional guidance. As both MTBI and PCS present with a constellation of cognitive, physical, and emotional symptoms, the reintroduction of physical activity must be tailored to each individual's specific needs and current state of health.

Gradual Integration of Exercise

The fundamental principle in reintroducing exercise after an MTBI or during the recovery from PCS is the gradual and monitored increase in physical activity. The brain's vulnerability post-injury necessitates a cautious approach to prevent exacerbation of symptoms and facilitate healing. Initiating with low-intensity activities and progressively increasing the intensity and duration, as tolerated, helps gauge the brain's capacity to handle physical exertion without triggering negative responses.

Monitoring Symptoms

A pivotal aspect of reintegrating exercise is vigilant symptom monitoring. Activities should be modified or halted at any sign of symptom exacerbation. This patient-centered approach ensures that exercise aids in recovery rather than impedes it. Symptoms to watch for include increased headache, dizziness, nausea, or a spike in cognitive disturbances such as memory or concentration difficulties.

The Role of Cardiovascular Exercise in Recovery

Cardiovascular exercise plays a critical role in the recovery process from MTBI and PCS for several reasons:

Increased Blood Flow to the Brain: Aerobic exercise promotes the circulation of blood throughout the body, including to the brain. This increased blood flow can aid in the healing process by delivering essential nutrients and oxygen to brain cells, supporting their recovery and function.

Neuroplasticity: Regular, moderate-intensity cardiovascular exercise has been shown to stimulate neuroplasticity—the brain's ability to form new neural connections. This process is crucial for recovery from brain injuries, as it underlies the brain's capacity to compensate for damaged areas and relearn lost functions.

Mood Regulation: Individuals recovering from MTBI and PCS often experience mood disturbances, including depression and anxiety. Cardiovascular exercise has well-documented benefits for mental health, including the reduction of stress and improvement of mood, partly due to the release of endorphins, often referred to as "feel-good" hormones.

Sleep Quality: Exercise can help regulate sleep patterns, which are often disrupted after a brain injury. Improved sleep quality is essential for brain healing and overall well-being.

Types of Cardiovascular Exercise Recommended

Given the need for caution, not all forms of cardiovascular exercise are suitable immediately following an MTBI or during PCS recovery. Recommended activities include:

Walking: Starting with short, gentle walks and gradually increasing the distance and pace as tolerated.

Stationary Cycling: Offers a controlled environment to exercise without the risk of falls or sudden head movements.

Swimming: Provides a low-impact option, though individuals should be symptom-free before engaging in swimming to avoid risks associated with water.

Conclusion

Incorporating cardiovascular exercise into the recovery plan for MTBI and PCS must be done judiciously, with the guidance of healthcare professionals who can tailor the exercise program to the individual's evolving needs. The benefits of cardiovascular exercise—enhanced brain function, mood regulation, improved sleep, and promotion of neuroplasticity — make it a vital component of the recovery process. However, the overarching principle should always be to listen to the body and adjust activities accordingly to ensure that exercise serves as a bridge to recovery, not a barrier.

The role of diet in concussion recovery

Adopting a nutritious diet following a concussion is a critical component of the recovery process, supporting the brain's healing and overall body health. Concussions, a form of mild traumatic brain injury (MTBI), can impact various bodily functions, including nutrient metabolism and appetite. Therefore, consulting with a healthcare professional or a registered dietitian to tailor a diet plan to your specific needs and symptoms is essential.

Principles of a Post-Concussion Diet

The objective of a post-concussion diet is to nourish the body and support brain health with balanced, nutrient-rich meals. Here's a guide to creating an effective dietary plan during recovery:

Balanced Meals and Snacks: Aim for three well-balanced meals and two to three healthy snacks per day. This helps maintain stable blood sugar levels, providing a constant energy supply to the brain and body.

Nutrient-Dense Foods: Focus on incorporating a variety of nutrient-dense foods into your diet. This includes:

Fruits and Vegetables: These are high in antioxidants, which can help reduce oxidative stress and inflammation in the brain.

Whole Grains: Foods like oats, quinoa, and whole wheat provide sustained energy and are rich in B vitamins, supporting brain function.

Lean Proteins: Sources such as chicken, fish, tofu, and legumes are essential for repair and growth of brain tissue.

Healthy Fats: Omega-3 fatty acids found in fish, flaxseeds, and walnuts are particularly beneficial for brain health, promoting neuronal healing and reducing inflammation.

Hydration: Staying adequately hydrated is crucial. Water is the best choice for hydration, but herbal teas and clear broths can also contribute to fluid intake. Proper hydration supports cognitive functions and helps in the transportation of nutrients to the brain.

Limit Processed and Sugary Foods: Reducing the intake of processed foods, sugary snacks, and beverages can help manage inflammation and promote better health outcomes. These foods can lead to spikes in blood sugar levels, affecting mood, energy, and overall recovery.

Adaptations for Eating Difficulties: Post-concussion, issues such as difficulty swallowing or decreased appetite can arise. Blending or pureeing foods can make eating easier and more appealing. For those needing to increase caloric and nutrient intake, consider fortified beverages or high-calorie supplements as part of your diet.

The Importance of Omega-3 Fatty Acids

Special emphasis should be placed on omega-3 fatty acids due to their significant benefits for brain health. They play a crucial role in repairing brain cells and reducing inflammation, which is paramount during the recovery from a concussion. Including omega-3-rich foods like fatty fish (salmon, mackerel, sardines), flaxseeds, and chia seeds can be particularly advantageous.

Implementing the Diet Plan

Implementing this diet plan requires mindfulness about food choices and listening to your body's signals. Recovery from a concussion varies from person to person, and so do dietary needs. Regular follow-ups with healthcare providers can help adjust the diet plan as recovery progresses, ensuring it meets changing nutritional requirements.

Conclusion

A well-structured, nutrient-dense diet plays a vital role in the recovery from a concussion, aiding in the restoration of brain function and overall well-being. By focusing on balanced meals, hydration, and the inclusion of specific nutrients beneficial for brain health, individuals can support their recovery journey effectively. Remember, personalization of the diet based on individual needs and professional advice is key to optimizing the recovery outcomes.

Chapter 17

Long-Term Effects

Long term impact of concussion and PCS

Most people who experience a concussion will fully recover within a few weeks or months. However, some people may experience long-term effects, such as:

Persistent symptoms

Some people may continue to experience symptoms, such as headache, dizziness, or difficulty with memory or concentration, long after the initial concussion.

Post-concussion syndrome

Post-concussion syndrome is a group of symptoms that can persist for weeks, months, or even years after a concussion. These symptoms may include headache, dizziness, fatigue, irritability, anxiety, and difficulty with memory and concentration.

Neurodegenerative conditions

In rare cases, a concussion may increase the risk of developing neurodegenerative conditions, such as dementia or Parkinson's disease.

Cognitive and behavioral problems

A concussion may cause changes in cognitive function, such as difficulty with memory or concentration, and may also lead to behavioral changes, such as irritability or difficulty with impulse control.

Increased risk of future concussions

People who have had a concussion are at increased risk of experiencing another one.

It is important to seek medical attention if you or someone you know experiences a concussion, especially if the person loses consciousness or experiences severe symptoms. Early diagnosis and treatment can help to prevent long-term complications and ensure a full recovery.

Epilepsy

Concussion can sometimes be followed by the development of epilepsy, which is a neurological disorder characterized by recurrent seizures. The exact cause of this link is not fully understood, but it is thought that the brain damage that occurs with concussion may increase the risk of developing epilepsy.

The risk of developing epilepsy after a concussion appears to be higher in individuals who have experienced more severe injuries or who have a history of brain injuries. The risk may also be increased in individuals who have other risk factors for epilepsy, such as a family history of the disorder or a pre-existing neurological condition. It is difficult to provide specific statistics on epilepsy after concussion, as the prevalence and incidence of epilepsy after concussion may vary depending on a number of factors, including the severity of the concussion, the patient's age and medical history, and other risk factors for epilepsy.

According to some studies, the risk of epilepsy after concussion may be higher in certain groups, such as children and adolescents, and may be more likely to occur in the first few years after the concussion. However, the overall risk of epilepsy after concussion is thought to be relatively low, with some estimates suggesting that the risk is less than 1%.

The symptoms of epilepsy can vary widely, and they may not always occur immediately after a concussion. Some individuals may experience seizures within a few days or weeks of the concussion, while others may not experience seizures for several months or even years after the injury.

Risk of stroke

There is evidence to suggest that individuals who have sustained a concussion may be at increased risk of experiencing a stroke. A stroke is a medical emergency that occurs when the blood supply to the brain is disrupted, resulting in brain damage and potentially permanent neurological deficits.

One possible mechanism through which concussion may increase the risk of stroke is through the development of cerebral microbleeds. These are small areas of bleeding in the brain that may occur as a result of trauma, such as a concussion. Microbleeds may increase the risk of stroke by disrupting the blood-brain barrier and causing inflammation in the brain.

Other factors that may increase the risk of stroke in individuals who have sustained a concussion include the presence of underlying medical conditions, such as hypertension or diabetes, and the use of certain medications, such as blood thinners.

It is important to note that the link between concussion and stroke risk is still being studied, and more research is needed to fully understand the relationship between these two conditions.

Concussion and chronic traumatic encephalopathy

Chronic traumatic encephalopathy (CTE) is a degenerative brain disease that can occur as a result of repeated head injuries, such as concussions. CTE is thought to be caused by a build-up of tau protein in the brain, which can lead to the death of brain cells and shrinkage of the brain.

CTE is most commonly associated with contact sports, such as football and boxing, as well as other activities that involve repeated head impacts, such as wrestling and martial arts. However, CTE can also occur as a result of other types of head injuries, such as those that occur in car accidents or falls.

Symptoms of CTE may not appear until years or even decades after the head injuries have occurred. These symptoms can include memory loss, confusion, impaired judgement, aggression, depression, and difficulty with balance and coordination. CTE can only be diagnosed after death, through an examination of the brain tissue.

It is important to take precautions to prevent head injuries and concussions, such as wearing protective gear when participating in sports or other high-energy activities, and seeking medical attention if you or someone you know experiences a concussion. Early diagnosis and treatment of a concussion can help to prevent long-term complications and ensure a full recovery.

Concussion and motor neuron disease

There is some evidence to suggest that concussion and other types of traumatic brain injury (TBI) may increase the risk of developing motor neuron disease (MND), which is a group of progressive neurological disorders that affect the motor neurons that control muscle movement.

MND is a rare condition, and the exact cause is not fully understood. It is thought to result from a combination of genetic and environmental factors. Some studies have suggested that TBI may contribute to the development of MND by causing inflammation and oxidative stress in the brain, which can lead to the death of neurons.

However, it is important to note that the link between concussion and MND is not fully understood, and more research is needed to confirm this association. The risk of developing MND after a concussion is thought to be low, and it is not known whether the risk is higher for individuals who have experienced multiple concussions or more severe injuries.

Parkinson's disease and concussion

There is some evidence to suggest that concussion and other types of traumatic brain injury (TBI) may increase the risk of developing Parkinson's disease (PD), a progressive neurological disorder that affects movement and is caused by the loss of dopamine-producing cells in the brain.

Several studies have found an increased risk of PD in individuals who have experienced TBI, particularly those who have experienced multiple injuries or more severe injuries. The exact mechanism by which TBI may increase the risk of PD is not fully understood, but it is thought to involve inflammation and oxidative stress in the brain, which can lead to the death of neurons.

However, it is important to note that the link between concussion and PD is not fully understood, and more research is needed to confirm this association. The risk of developing PD after a concussion is thought to be low, and it is not known whether the risk is higher for individuals who have experienced multiple concussions or more severe injuries.

Strategies for managing and minimizing long-term effects

There are several strategies that can help to manage and minimize the long-term effects of concussion:

Seek medical attention

It is important to seek medical attention if you or someone you know experiences a concussion, especially if the person loses consciousness or experiences severe symptoms. Early diagnosis and treatment can help to prevent long-term complications and ensure a full recovery.

Follow treatment recommendations

Follow the recommended treatment plan, including rest and time, medication, and rehabilitation as needed, to support recovery from a concussion.

Avoid high-risk activities

To minimize the risk of future concussions, it may be necessary to avoid high-risk activities, such as contact sports or other activities that involve high speeds or impacts.

Use protective gear

Wearing protective gear, such as a helmet or other protective headwear, can help to reduce the risk of concussion in activities that carry a risk of head injury.

Manage persistent symptoms

If you continue to experience symptoms, such as headache, dizziness, or difficulty with memory or concentration, after a concussion, it is important to work with a healthcare provider to manage these symptoms and minimize their impact on your daily life.

By following these strategies, you can help to manage and minimize the long-term effects of concussion and ensure a full recovery.

Ways to reduce the risk of concussion

There are several ways to reduce the risk of concussion, including:

Wear protective gear

Wearing protective gear, such as a helmet or other protective headwear, can help to reduce the risk of concussion in activities that carry a risk of head injury.

Follow safety guidelines

Follow safety guidelines and rules when participating in sports or other high-energy activities to reduce the risk of concussion.

Use caution when engaging in physical activities

Be cautious when engaging in physical activities, such as skateboarding or snowboarding, and use protective gear to reduce the risk of concussion.

Avoid substance abuse

Substance abuse, including alcohol abuse, can increase the risk of concussion. Avoiding substance abuse can help to reduce the risk of concussion.

Supervise children

Supervise young children to prevent falls and other accidents that could lead to concussion.

By following these guidelines and taking precautions, you can help to reduce the risk of concussion and protect yourself and others from this type of brain injury.

Importance of proper management and care to prevent further injury

Proper management and care after a concussion is important to prevent further injury and ensure a full recovery. This may include:

Rest and time: Taking a break from physical and mental activity, including sports and other high-energy activities, and getting plenty of sleep can help to support recovery from a concussion.

Medication

Over-the-counter pain medications, such as acetaminophen (Tylenol) or ibuprofen (Advil), can be used to manage headache and other pain symptoms.

Rehabilitation

Physical therapy or other rehabilitation techniques can help with balance and coordination and support recovery from a concussion.

Follow-up care

It is important to follow up with a healthcare provider after experiencing a concussion to ensure that symptoms are improving and to monitor for any long-term complications.

Proper management and care can help to prevent further injury and ensure a full recovery from a concussion. If you or someone you know has experienced a concussion, it is important to seek medical attention and follow the recommended treatment plan.

Chapter 18

Finding resources and support groups

Concussion support groups

There are a number of resources and support groups available for people with concussions and their loved ones. Here are some tips for finding support groups and other resources:

Talk to your healthcare provider

Your healthcare provider can be a valuable resource for finding support groups and other resources for people with concussions. They may have information about local support groups or be able to refer you to other resources.

Search online

There are many online resources and support groups available for people with concussions. A simple online search can yield a range of options, such as online support groups, forums, and information about local support groups

Contact a concussion advocacy organization There are organizations that advocate for people with concussions and their families and may be able to provide information about support groups and other resources. Some examples of concussion advocacy organizations include the Concussion Legacy Foundation and the Brain Injury Association of America.

Contact a local brain injury organization

Many local brain injury organizations offer support groups and other resources for people with concussions and their families. A simple online search or a call to a local hospital can yield information about these organizations.

Headway is a charity organization in the United Kingdom that provides support and services to people affected by brain injury, as well as their families and caregivers. The organization was founded in 1979, and has since become a leading provider of support and information on brain injury in the UK. Headway offers a wide range of services and support to people affected by brain injury, including rehabilitation, residential care, community support, and education and training. The organization also provides information and resources on brain injury, including information on the causes and effects of brain injury, and guidance on how to manage and cope with brain injury. Headway's website, headway.org, is a comprehensive resource for information on brain injury, and includes information on the organization's services and support, as well as resources for individuals affected by brain injury and their families and caregivers. The website also includes information on brain injury research, advocacy, and fundraising initiatives.

Overall, there are many resources and support groups available for people with concussions and their loved ones. It is important to seek out these resources and find the support that works best for you.

Chapter 19

Concussion rules in contact sports

Concussion rules in Rugby

In rugby, a concussion is a common injury that can occur as a result of contact to the head or neck. Concussions can have serious short-term and long-term effects, so it's important that they are managed properly to ensure the safety of players.

There are several rules in place to help manage and prevent concussions in rugby. These include:

Head injury assessment (HIA)

This is a procedure that involves a team doctor evaluating a player who has sustained a head injury or concussion during a match. The player must leave the field of play if the HIA is positive.

Return to play protocol

This is a step-by-step process that a player must follow after sustaining a concussion. The player must pass each step before being cleared to return to play.

Tackle height

In some versions of rugby, there are rules in place that aim to reduce the risk of head and neck injuries by limiting the height at which players can tackle each other.

Foul play

Players who intentionally cause head injuries or concussions through foul play can be penalized or suspended.

It's important to note that these rules may vary depending on the level of play and the specific governing body. It's also important to remember that concussions can occur as a result of other types of impacts besides tackles, such as collisions with other players or the ground.

Concussion rules in boxing

In boxing, a concussion is a common injury that can occur as a result of blows to the head. Concussions can have serious short-term and long-term effects, so it's important that they are managed properly to ensure the safety of boxers.

There are several rules in place to help manage and prevent concussions in boxing. These include

Medical examination

Before a boxing match, a doctor will typically perform a medical examination to ensure that the boxers are healthy and fit to compete. This may include checking for any signs of a previous concussion or head injury.

Boxers are required to wear headgear and mouthguards to help protect against concussions and other head injuries.

Stoppages

If a boxer is knocked down or appears to be injured, the referee can stop the fight to allow the boxer to be examined by a doctor. If the doctor determines that the boxer is unable to continue, the fight can be stopped.

Suspensions

If a boxer sustains a concussion or other head injury during a fight, they may be required to take time off to recover before being allowed to return to the ring.

It's important to note that these rules may vary depending on the specific governing body and the level of competition. It's also important to remember that concussions can occur as a result of other types of impacts besides punches, such as falls to the canvas or collisions with the ropes.

Chapter 20

Recap of key points

Take-home points

Concussion is a type of brain injury that occurs when the brain is jarred or shaken inside the skull.

Concussions are common, especially in children and adolescents who are active in sports and other high-energy activities.

The impact of a concussion can vary widely, depending on the severity of the injury and the individual's age, health, and other factors.

Common causes of concussion include falls, sports and physical activity, traffic accidents, physical violence, blast injuries, and shaken baby syndrome.

Risk factors for concussion include age, participation in sports and other high-energy activities, previous concussions, substance abuse, and certain medical conditions.

Common symptoms of concussion include headache, dizziness, confusion, memory problems, nausea and vomiting, fatigue, sensitivity to light and noise, sleep disturbances, and mood changes.

Diagnostic tools and techniques for concussion include physical examination, neurological examination, neuroimaging, balance and coordination tests, and symptom checklists.

Treatment options for concussion may include rest and time, over-the-counter pain medications, physical therapy, and hospitalization or surgery in more severe cases.

Proper management and care, including rest and time, medication, rehabilitation, and follow-up care, can help to prevent long-term complications and ensure a full recovery from a concussion.

In rare cases, a concussion may lead to long-term complications, such as persistent symptoms, post-concussion syndrome, neurodegenerative conditions, cognitive and behavioral problems, and an increased risk of future concussions.

Strategies for managing and minimizing the long-term effects of concussion include seeking medical attention, following treatment recommendations, avoiding high-risk activities, using protective gear, and managing persistent symptoms.

Ways to reduce the risk of concussion include wearing protective gear, following safety guidelines, using caution when engaging in physical activities, avoiding substance abuse, and supervising children.

Proper management and care after a concussion, including rest and time, medication, rehabilitation, and follow-up care, can help to prevent further injury and ensure a full recovery.

Concussions can be life changing injuries

It is important to take concussion seriously and seek proper care and treatment to prevent long-term complications and ensure a full recovery. Concussion is a type of brain injury that can have serious consequences if left untreated.

If you or someone you know experiences a concussion, it is important to seek medical attention as soon as possible. Symptoms of a concussion can range from mild to severe, and may not always be immediately apparent. Early diagnosis and treatment can help to prevent long-term complications and ensure a full recovery.

To reduce the risk of concussion, it is important to take precautions, such as wearing protective gear when participating in sports or other high-energy activities, and avoiding substance abuse. By following these guidelines, you can help to protect yourself and others from concussion and ensure a full recovery if a concussion does occur.

Emphasis on the importance of prevention and ongoing management to support recovery and prevent long-term complications.

Prevention and ongoing management are important to support recovery and prevent long-term complications of concussion. To reduce the risk of concussion, it is important to take precautions, such as wearing protective gear when participating in sports or other high-energy activities, and avoiding substance abuse.

If you or someone you know experiences a concussion, it is important to seek medical attention as soon as possible and follow the recommended treatment plan. This may include rest and time, medication, rehabilitation, and follow-up care. By following these guidelines, you can help to prevent further injury and ensure a full recovery.

Ongoing management and care are also important to prevent long-term complications of concussion. This may include avoiding high-risk activities, using protective gear, and managing persistent symptoms. By taking these steps, you can help to minimize the long-term effects of concussion and ensure a full recovery.